THE DIET COOKBOOK FOR MENOPAUSE

A Complete Guide on Menopause with 20-Healthy

Delicious Recipes to Manage Your Symptoms

TABLE OF CONTENT

INTRODUCTION

Menopause shouldn't be a secret or mystery, and you shouldn't have to put up with it in silence This smorgasbord of symptoms, which can impact careers, relationships and quality of life can be particularly severe sometimes to some than other. But it's important to recognize what your body needs long term and not ignore the changes if they occur.

It's useful to remember that menopause is not a disease and even a difficult transition will eventually settle down. Perimenopause may be rocky or tumultuous because it's a time of change but on the other side most studies report that women who've gone through that change in the hormones are now not on that crazy up-and-down rollercoaster ride. Know that most symptoms will go away, and you will see the light at the end of the tunnel.

Meanwhile, several lifestyle factors can help you mitigate the physical and psychological impacts of menopause and even empower it and you can start embracing this inevitable life change.

it's time for attitudes to change, we need to start recognizing menopause as a natural part of life and an opportunity to reinvent one's life, relationships, and future goals with renewed vigour. You can also optimize your health earlier. If you arrive at menopause at that transition time and you're healthy, you've got a good diet, you don't get too stressed, you're probably going to have less symptoms. But it's never too late to start turning things around.

Menopause is when you stop having periods. Menopause means the last menstrual period. Know that it's not only those who identify as women who will experience menopause. Some transgender men, non-binary people and intersex people or people with variations in sex characteristics may also experience menopause. Menopause is a natural event and transition that you will experience, however, the timing and symptoms are different for everyone.

You can look at your family history to get an idea of when you might go through it. It's likely to be a similar age to when your mother or older sisters started theirs. Also menopause can also occur due to certain surgeries or cancer treatments. This can sometimes cause symptoms to be more sudden and in some cases more severe.

Menopause usually happens between the ages of 45 and 55. Your genetics play a role in when you will experience menopause, as many women start around the same age as their mothers. Other factors that can affect when you start menopause include smoking, cancer treatment, and the surgical removal of the ovaries. During menopause, your ovaries slow down the production of estrogen and progesterone which result in the following symptoms; Bone density loss., Difficulty sleeping, Dry skin, Hair loss, Hot flashes and night sweats, Joint pain, Mood swings, depression, and irritability and lot more.

CHAPTER ONE

MENOPAUSE PREP

Menopause is divided into three basic stages: perimenopause, menopause, and postmenopause. During this time, the ovaries begin to atrophy which causes a decline in the production of the hormones that stimulate the menstrual cycle; estrogen and progesterone. Additionally, as you age there is a natural decline in the number of eggs in the ovaries. As a result, fertility declines. The transition from perimenopause to menopause to post-menopause usually lasts seven years or longer. Understanding the stages will help you know what to expect, how to better manage your symptoms, and know when it's time to talk to your healthcare provider.

PERIMENOPAUSE

The perimenopause or pre-menopause stage occurs about three to five years before menopause. The age at which you start experiencing this stage can vary greatly. Although, most females begins to experience symptoms in their mid to late forties.

It is rare to notice symptoms prior to age 40. During this stage, your estrogen and progesterone levels begin to fluctuate. You may begin to experience mood changes, irregular menstrual cycles and other menopausal symptoms. During this stage, it's still possible to get pregnant, so continuing a form of birth control is important.

MENOPAUSE

Menopause is defined as the absence of menses for 12 straight months without other causes, such as illness, medication or pregnancy. Once you reach menopause, you can no longer achieve pregnancy.

The average age of menopause is 51, but the age can vary greatly. Some enter this stage in their mid-forties and others not until mid-fifties.

POST-MENOPAUSE

The post-menopause stage signals the end of your reproductive years. While your ovaries produce low levels of estrogen and progesterone, you no longer will ovulate or menstruate. Once you enter the post-menopause stage, you're in it for the rest of your life.

You may continue to have the same symptoms you experienced during the perimenopause and menopause stages for many years after your final menstrual cycle. Fortunately, these symptoms tend to dissipate over time. However, females in this stage are at an increased risk of heart disease and osteoporosis due to the decrease in estrogen.

The good news is no matter which stage you find yourself in, menopause symptoms often can be managed by a healthy diet, regular exercise and lifestyle modifications.

However, if your symptoms are intense enough to disrupt your quality of life, then it's time to talk to your gynecologist or healthcare provider.

Together, you can develop a personalized care plan, which may include hormone replacement therapy or other medications that will control your symptoms and improve daily function.

Menopause is manageable. In fact, many report it as a positive step into a new stage in life.

HOW TO RELIEVE MENOPAUSE SYMPTOMS

There is no way to avoid menopause but you can survive and thrive during this change and experience menopause on your own terms by learning ways to relieve your symptoms and definitely why you are reading this book to teach you how and definitely I will teach you.

- Of the many lifestyle factors that can help deal with menopause and protect against long-term health problems, exercise is fundamental. Falling oestrogen levels impact bone density, making bones more vulnerable to fracture. Muscle mass and strength decline with age, which can slow metabolism and cause muscle tissue to be replaced by fat. The hormonal changes during menopause also shift fat distribution from the hips to the stomach area, bringing greater risk of heart disease and diabetes. The best way to strengthen bones and maintain muscle mass is through weight-bearing exercises, such as resistance or strength training. But you don't need fancy gym equipment.

- Ageing itself can increase weight unless lifestyle factors are addressed. On top of that, oestrogen helps with insulin sensitivity, so declining levels can bring greater risk of diabetes. Considering this, it's more important than ever to be mindful of eating a healthy diet that is low in sugar and refined carbohydrates. To mitigate weight gain and diabetes risk, the importance of eating less carbs and more protein. Falling oestrogen levels can also increase blood pressure and unhealthy cholesterol levels. Ultimately, increased exercise and nutritious diet together are vital to tip the scales in favour of maintaining a healthy weight and avoiding chronic disease at this life stage more than ever. Other considerations include extra calcium and vitamin D to support bone health, and if necessary, reducing alcohol intake to ease hot flushes and promote better sleep. There is also increasing evidence that avoiding processed foods, sugar, alcohol and caffeine can reduce symptoms like hot flushes or night sweats even menopause migraines.

- Hormone replacement therapy (or menopause replacement therapy (MRT) as it's now known) with bio-identical hormones is not a stand-alone treatment, but it can help. It generally has more benefits than it has risks. This doesn't mean trying to achieve pre-menopausal hormone levels; it is most useful for relieving the more severe symptoms. The aim of the treatment is never to replace the hormones to the level that they were when you were 25 years old. This therapy is not for all. For instance, those who have had breast cancer, smoke or are overweight. But mostly it important for you to have an individualized treatment plan with a health professional to weigh up the risks and benefits. And don't feel that HRT is a magic bullet and that it will relieve all your symptoms. A holistic approach is required to properly manage menopause long term.

- Our skin doesn't escape the impacts of falling hormone levels, compounding the effects of ageing. For some, it's just dry skin; for others, it can be worse. During perimenopause your skin can start to change. Have heard different stories on how my clients complain about their skin; Decreased oestrogen can also impact the skin's collagen levels, contributing to ageing skin and wrinkling. Avoiding tobacco, limiting sun exposure and adequate sleep all play a role in skin health, as well as keeping it moisturised and eating a healthy diet.

- Stress, stress, stress is a major factor. Our modern days are so full, we are looking after families, often caring for aged relatives and trying to earn a living. It doesn't help that changing hormones can affect sleep quality, which is also disrupted by night sweats. Good sleep habits or "sleep hygiene" can help, such as going to bed and getting up at a regular time, relaxing away from screens and avoiding caffeine or a full stomach before bedtime. Fluctuating hormones, along with poor sleep, can contribute to depression and anxiety in some women. Exercise, healthy diet and calming activities such as yoga and meditation can help manage these issues. It's also a good time to nurture friendships and take time out to care for yourself, seeking help when it's all too much.

Going through menopause does not have to affect your overall quality of life. Menopause is just another adjustment you need to make in their lifetime, we can use menopause as a time for reflection and reclaim this as a powerful life stage when you can eventually feel liberated and empowered. But you don't need to go through it alone there's help and I would love to see you as you embrace and revered at this time of your live with my book.

THE MENOPAUSE MANAGEMENT STRATEGIES

Foods to Eat During Menopause and Beyond

The menopause can be a difficult time and I could understand why many are drawn to the idea of supplements or changing their diet to help. But still yet I know you still cycle around the question that; is there any evidence to back any of the claims? Can anything help with symptoms? Can changes you make to your diet help with your long-term health? Yes! There are evidence behind all this and you are about to discover that.

- Reducing caffeine, alcohol and spicy food in your diet may help hot flushes, but there is considerable variation between individuals. Current recommended limits of alcohol are a total of 14 units a week, with a maximum of two per day. Reducing alcohol also has other health benefits, such as a lower risk of liver disease, heart disease, osteoporosis, type 2 diabetes, and certain types of cancer such as breast cancer.

- For some women insomnia can be a symptom of the menopause. Unfortunately, there is very little evidence to support any benefit from magnesium supplements. Instead you should be able to meet all your magnesium needs through a healthy diet containing wholegrains, spinach, pumpkin seeds, almonds and beans.

- Phytoestrogens are plant derived compounds, that have a similar structure to human estrogen, and similar but weaker activity. They are found in foods and in a more concentrated form in supplements. Phytoestrogens supplements are frequently marketed and chosen to target hot flushes

There are a number of herbal medicines that contain phytoestrogens that may help with the symptoms of menopause.

There is evidence to support decreased hot flushes with St John's wort, black cohosh, and genistein.

Declining levels of estrogen from the menopause and beyond increases your risk of cardiovascular disease (heart disease and strokes) and osteoporosis (brittle bones and increased risk of fractures), diabetes, depression, obesity and dementia. If you experience early or premature menopause, your risk is unfortunately higher. To counteract these concerns you can make some dietary changes to reduce your long-term risks.

Osteoporosis leads to a greater risk of having low energy fractures. Estrogen has a really important role in bone health, and as levels decline, risk of osteoporosis increases. A 50 year old woman only has a 2% risk of osteoporosis, compared with a 25% risk in an 80 year old lady, due to considerably lower levels of estrogen. Diet can play an important role in bone health.

There are some key macronutrients, vitamins and minerals to be sure that you are getting enough of:

- Quality protein: Include lean protein foods at every meal such as seafood, beans, legumes, dairy, meat, and poultry.

- Calcium is an important mineral for bone health, and as an adult before the menopause you need to 700mg per day while from the menopause this rises to 1200mg a day. Good sources of calcium include dairy, calcium-fortified plant-based drinks, tinned fish (with bones), spinach, fortified bread, baked beans, tofu and dried figs. If you are unable to have enough in your diet, you might be prescribed a supplement.

- Vitamin D, commonly called the sunshine vitamin as it is produced by the action of sunlight on our skin during exposure outside. Current NHS guidance is for women to consider taking a supplement of 10mcg

(400IU) during the autumn and winter months as it can be difficult to get enough sun exposure. Vitamin D is also found in low levels egg yolks, oily fish and some fortified foods, but is difficult to get enough from diet alone. It was previously thought that sunscreen prevented vitamin D formation, but evidence suggests that sunscreen does not inhibit vitamin D production in the skin.

- The term vitamin K covers a number of different molecules and you need to eat a range of items to ensure you get all the different elements. Vitamin K is found in green vegetables, fermented food, dairy, and meat and has an important role in bone strength. Although there is mixed evidence as to whether vitamin K supplementation improves bone strength and reduces fractures, a number of countries for example Japan, now include vitamin K supplementation as treatment for osteoporosis. Vitamin K is a fat-soluble vitamin, and is stored if you take excess. It is therefore possible to have too much through supplementation, and we don't know what these effects might be. If you are on blood thinning medication, you should avoid taking vitamin K supplements as they can interfere.

- Phosphorus is found in foods such as poultry, meat, dairy, oily fish, potatoes, wholegrains, pulses and beans. It is usually abundant in our diet, and you should not need to take a supplement.

- Magnesium is another mineral that is usually abundant in our diet but good sources include wholegrains, spinach, pumpkin seeds, almonds and beans. Again you should not need to supplement this.

PRACTICAL TIPS FOR OPTIMIZING YOUR DIET

The menopause is a time of immense change, with you experiencing a spectrum of severity of symptoms. Dietary changes might not be possible for you right away, but try to incorporate them where possible for long-term health benefits. Aim to eat a variety of colours, whole grains, quality protein at every meal, unsaturated fats, whole plant-based foods, items rich in calcium and optimize your gut health.

Ultimately the best way to support a healthy weight, reduced long-term risk of cardiovascular disease and osteoporosis is by regular exercise and a healthy diet that follows these principles:

- Eat lots of different coloured fruit and vegetables.

- Choose wholegrains (bulgur wheat, millet, sweet potatoes, brown rice, brown bread).

- Eat a handful of nuts a day and add seeds to your food.

- Eat oily fish twice a week. If you do not eat fish, have daily nuts, and seeds which also contain omega 3.

- Chose lean or plant-based protein at every meal.

- Regularly enjoy beans, lentils and chickpeas.

- Enjoy healthy unsaturated fats such avocados, rapeseed, nuts and extra virgin olive oils.

- Aim for a handful of nuts and seeds a day.

- Avoid convenience products that have high amounts of sugar and salt, and sugary fizzy drinks.

- Avoid sweeteners.

- Support your microbiota to flourish by eating fermented foods, kefir, and 30g of fibre a day.

- Try to reduce alcohol, and try to keep less than 14 units of alcohol per week (maximum of 2 units per day).

- Enjoy lots of calcium rich foods (1200mg per day from the menopause onwards).

CHAPTER TWO

RECIPES FOR MENOPAUSE

Spinach Omelette

Total Time: 10 Minutes

Ingredients

- 1 cup spinach leaves

- 2 cloves garlic

- 2 eggs

- 1 tablespoon milk skimmed optional

- Salt to taste

- 1 teaspoon olive oil

- 2 tablespoon Parmesan cheese grated

- 1/2 teaspoon chilli flakes optional for seasoning

Directions

- Prep the ingredients. Wash and chop the spinach leaves. Don't let the leaves go dry. Leave some water. Thinly slice the garlic. Crack the eggs into a bowl, and add a tablespoon of milk. Add a pinch of salt, and whisk the eggs gently just enough for the yolk to mix well.

- Heat a cast iron skillet (or any other frying pan), and add the chopped spinach, garlic, and sprinkle some salt. Let the leaves wilt, and take them off the skillet.

- Pour a teaspoon olive oil on the pan, and spread it evenly with a spatula. Reduce the flame to medium, and pour the egg mixture. Tilt the pan and let the eggs spread evenly. As soon as the omelette start to set, lift near the edges with the spatula so that the uncooked eggs can reach the bottom of the pan. Once the center starts to set, top half of the omelette with the cooked spinach and garlic. Now sprinkle the grated cheese on top of it.

- Lower the flame, and cook further. Wait for the cheese to start melting, and once the omelette starts to get detached from sides, fold in half. Gently slide the omelette to a plate.

Sour Cream and Green Onion Scrambled Eggs

Total Time: 15 Minutes

Ingredients

- 8 large eggs

- 1 ¼ cup whole milk

- 2 tablespoon sour cream

- ¼ cup shaved or shredded Parmesan cheese

- 3 tablespoon sliced green onion

- 1 tablespoon butter

- ½ teaspoon salt

- ½ teaspoon black pepper

Directions

- Crack eggs into a medium mixing bowl. Add milk, sour cream, salt, and pepper. Whisk till combined and pale yellow. There should be a few air bubbles formed on the surface from whisking.

- In a medium rimmed skillet, heat butter over medium-low heat. Add the eggs and sprinkle green onions on top.

- Allow sides of the eggs to loosely set and pull in the sides to form the scrambled eggs.

- When eggs are about half done (still runny, but forming solids), add the Parmesan to the eggs. Keep pulling in the sides of the eggs till eggs are set and cheese is partially melted.

- Remove from heat, serve, and enjoy with a glass of milk and buttered toast.

Sesame Bean Sprouts Salad

Total Time: 6 Minutes

Ingredients

- 4-5 cups bean sprouts

- 4 teaspoons low sodium soy sauce

- 4 teaspoons sesame oil

- 1 teaspoon toasted sesame seeds

- 2 cloves garlic, minced

- 3-4 stalks green onions, finely sliced

Directions

- Add enough water to a pot to cover the bean sprouts. Do not add the bean sprouts yet though! Bring the pot of water to a full boil.

- In the meantime, wash the bean sprouts very well by transferring them to a large bowl and filling the bowl with cold water. Vigorously swish the sprout with your hand to rinse them well. Drain off the water and repeat. Do this until the water runs completely clear!

- Once the pot of water is boiling, add the bean sprouts to the pot and blanch for 1 minute.

- Remove the bean sprouts from the boiling water immediately and immerse them in a bowl of cold water. Cool the blanched bean sprouts completely and drain well.

- Next, in a mixing bowl, whisk together the soy sauce, sesame oil, sesame seeds, garlic, and green onions.

- Add the bean sprouts and toss to coat.

- You can eat the salad immediately, or you can let it set at room temperature for 15-20 minutes first if you prefer not to have a cold salad. Alternatively, for maximum flavour, cover and refrigerate for one hour before serving. This allows the flavours time to come together and to be honest, this side salad is best served chilled.

Roasted Brussels Sprouts Quinoa Salad

Total Time: 20 Minutes

Ingredients

- 1 lb. Brussels sprouts, ends trimmed and halved (or quartered, if large)

- 3 garlic cloves, minced

- 1 tablespoon avocado oil or olive oil

- ⅓ cup pecans, chopped and toasted

- ¼ cup dried cranberries or dried cherries

- ¼ cup shaved Parmesan cheese

- ½ cup uncooked quinoa

- 1 cup water

- 2 tablespoons olive oil

- Juice of ½ orange

- ½ teaspoon orange zest

- 2 teaspoon apple cider vinegar

- 1 teaspoon Dijon mustard

- 1 teaspoon pure maple syrup

- 1 teaspoon fresh thyme leaves (or ½ teaspoon dried thyme)

- Fine salt and black pepper to taste

Directions

- Preheat the oven to 400°F.

- On a sheet pan, combine the Brussels sprouts and minced garlic. Toss with 1 tablespoon olive oil and sprinkle with salt and pepper. Arrange the Brussels so they are all cut-side down on the baking sheet (Tip: This helps them roast better and get more evenly browned).

- Roast in the oven until Brussels sprouts are tender and golden brown, 15-20 minutes.

- While the Brussels sprouts are roasting, in a small saucepan, bring 1 cup of water plus a pinch of salt to a boil. Once the water is boiling, add the quinoa and stir. Reduce the heat to a simmer, cover, and continue to cook for 15 minutes or until quinoa is tender and liquid is absorbed. Remove pan from heat and let set for 10-15 minutes covered.

- While the Brussels sprouts and quinoa are cooking, in a small bowl, combine the 2 tablespoons olive oil, orange juice, zest, vinegar, mustard, maple syrup, and thyme; whisk to combine. Season with salt and pepper to taste.

- In a serving dish, combine the roasted Brussels sprouts, cooked quinoa, toasted pecans, and dried cranberries. Pour the vinaigrette on all and gently toss to combine. Sprinkle with Parmesan cheese. Serve warm or cold.

- Store leftovers in an airtight container in the fridge for up to 3 days.

Crispy Artichoke White Bean Salad

Total Time: 25 Minutes

Ingredients

- 15 oz can quartered artichoke hearts, packed in water or brine

- 2 teaspoons olive oil

- Juice of half a lemon

- 1 tablespoon grated Parmesan cheese

- Kosher salt and pepper, to taste

- 1/4 cup olive oil

- 2 to 3 tablespoons lemon juice

- 1 tablespoon champagne vinegar

- 2 teaspoons honey

- 1 teaspoon Dijon mustard

- 1 clove garlic, minced

- Kosher salt and pepper, to taste

- 1 small head green cabbage, thinly sliced and chopped

- 1 cucumber finely diced

- 15 oz white beans, rinsed and drained

- 3 green onions sliced

- 1/2 cup chopped basil

- 1/2 cup freshly grated Parmesan cheese

- 1/4 cup chopped Italian parsley

- Kosher salt and black pepper, to taste

Directions

- Preheat the oven to 400 degrees.

- Drain the artichokes and place them on paper towels. Gently press on the artichokes to squeeze out as much liquid as possible. Pat dry with paper towels. Place the artichokes on a large baking sheet. Drizzle with olive oil and toss. Space the artichokes out so they aren't touching. Squeeze the lemon over the top and sprinkle with parmesan cheese. Season with salt and pepper. Place in the oven and roast for 10 to 15 minutes or until crispy. Alternatively, you can use the air fryer.

- While the artichokes are roasting, make the dressing. In a small bowl, whisk together the olive oil, lemon juice, vinegar, honey, mustard, garlic, salt, and pepper. Set aside.

- In a large bowl, combine the cabbage, cucumber, white beans, green onions, basil, Parmesan cheese, parsley, and roasted artichokes. Toss well. Drizzle the dressing over the salad and toss again until salad is well coated. Taste and season with salt and pepper, to taste. Serve.

Beet Salad with Feta

Total Time: 25 Minutes

Ingredients

- 6 ounces Fresh Spinach

- 6 Cooked Beets sliced

- ½ cup Feta

- 1 tablespoon Green Onions sliced

- 1 teaspoon Extra-virgin olive oil

- 1 tablespoon Balsamic Glaze

Directions

- Place the fresh spinach in a large bowl.

- Slice the cooked beets and place on top of the spinach.

- Then sprinkle on feta and sliced green onions. Drizzle olive oil and balsamic reduction and serve.

Cinnamon raisin quinoa granola

Total Time: 50 Minutes

Ingredients

- 2 cups raw quinoa (any type)

- 1 cup coconut flakes

- ½ cup ground walnuts

- 2 tsp cinnamon

- ¼ cup brown sugar

- ¼ tsp salt

- ⅓ cup chopped walnuts

- 1 tbsp honey or maple syrup

- ¼ cup vegetable oil

- ½ cup vanilla almond milk

- 1 tsp vanilla extract

- Add after baking:

- ⅓ cup raisins

- ⅓ cup cranberries

Directions

- Pre-heat oven to 275 F. Line a large baking sheet with parchment paper

- In a large bowl, combine dry ingredients. Set aside

- In a small bowl, combine wet ingredients and mix well

- Add the wet ingredients to dry.

- Mix well using your hands, so the quinoa is coated evenly.

- Spread evenly on lined baking sheet, to form one thin, single layer (you may need to bake it in two batches)

- Bake for 30 minutes at 275F, checking and mixing every 15 minutes so it cooks evenly. Turn off the oven and leave the granola inside the oven until it cools.

- Remove granola from the oven and add raisins and cranberries. Mix well

- Let it cool completely and store in an airtight container

Total Time: 2 Hours

Ingredients

- 1 1/2 cups old-fashioned rolled oats

- 1 cup milk

- 1 cup all-purpose flour

- 1 teaspoon baking powder

- 1 teaspoon ground cinnamon

- 1/2 teaspoon baking soda

- 1/2 teaspoon kosher salt

- 1/2 cup (1 stick) unsalted butter, melted and cooled

- 2 large eggs, lightly beaten

- 1/2 cup lightly packed brown sugar

- 1/4 cup diced dried apricots

- 1/3 cup white chocolate chips

- 1/4 cup dried cranberries

Directions

- Combine the oats and milk in a large bowl and let stand 30 minutes.

- Preheat the oven to 400 degrees F. Line 10 cups of a 12-cup muffin tin with paper liners

- In a separate medium bowl, whisk together the flour, baking powder, cinnamon, baking soda and salt.

- Stir the melted butter, eggs and brown sugar into the bowl of oats and milk until well combined. Stir the flour mixture into the oat mixture until well combined. Fold in the white chocolate chips and dried apricots.

- Using an ice-cream scoop or 2 large tablespoons, divide the batter among the 10 lined muffin tins. Bake until a toothpick inserted into the center of a muffin comes out with some crumbs sticking to it, about 20 minutes. Let the muffins cool 5 minutes in the tins before removing them to a wire rack to cool completely.

Poached Eggs With Avocado and Feta Smash on Sourdough

Total Time: 25 Minutes

Ingredients

- 1 large ripe avocado, peeled and halved

- 1 tablespoon lemon juice

- 60g crumbled feta cheese, goat or cow milk

- 2 tablespoons chopped parsley

- 1 tablespoon chopped dill

- 100g cherry tomatoes, chopped

- 8 eggs

- 1 tablespoon white vinegar

- 8 thick slices sourdough bread

Directions

- Place avocado halves in a bowl, fork through to create a rustic mash

- Add lemon juice, crumbled feta, chopped parsley, dill and tomato. Mix well

- Bring a medium shallow saucepan of water and vinegar to the boil. Break egg into a small dish and keep aside

- Reduce the heat and bring water to a simmer. Carefully slide in the egg

- Break remaining eggs into small dish one by one, and add to water

- Allow 3-4 minutes for poached eggs with firm whites and soft runny yolks. Cook longer for a firmer egg. Remove with a slotted spoon, rest on a paper towel to absorb any excess water

- Smear avocado smash on toasted sourdough and top with poached eggs

Banana Fritters

Total Time: 15 Minutes

Ingredients

- 1 cup all purpose or cake flour

- 1 teaspoon baking powder

- pinch salt

- ⅓ cup brown or white granulated sugar

- 3 ripe bananas mashed

- Vegetable oil, canola or sunflower oil for frying

- 1 teaspoon ground cinnamon

- ¼ cup brown sugar

Directions

- Sift the flour and baking powder into a bowl. Add the sugar and mix in the mashed bananas to form a sticky batter.

- Heat oil, to 356F /180°C in a deep fryer or heavy bottomed pan See note 1

- When hot, drop in teaspoonful of the batter and fry until golden brown about one minute on each side.

- Remove the fritters from the oil and drain on kitchen paper. Roll the fritters in the cinnamon sugar mixture before serving.

- Mix the cinnamon sugar ingredients together until well combined.

Vegan Tofu Scramble with Veggies

Total Time: 25 Minutes

Ingredients

- 2 tablespoons of cooking oil

- 1 small red bell pepper diced

- ½ of a yellow onion diced

- 1 garlic clove minced

- 1 (16-ounce) package of firm tofu

- 2 cups of baby spinach (optional)

- 1 cup of polenta (optional)

- 2 tablespoons of vegan margarine

- 1 tablespoon of turmeric

- 1 tablespoon of nutritional yeast (optional)

- 1 teaspoon of oregano

- Salt and pepper, to taste

Directions

- In a large frying pan, cook the bell pepper, onions, and garlic in most of the cooking oil for a few minutes.

- Crumble the tofu using your fingers into the pan and stir it up.

- If you are using polenta (it really makes it wet, like scrambled eggs, but we only use this recipe when we have leftover polenta) add this in and stir the mixture.

- Next, add the spinach, and vegan margarine, let it melt, and stir so that it is coating the tofu crumbles. Add in the turmeric and nutritional yeast (optional) and once again stir.

- Add in most of your veggies. If you are using veggies that cook longer such as broccoli, carrots, or potatoes you want to let them cook for about 10 minutes before adding in veggies that cook fast including mushrooms, kale, spinach, and tomatoes. You should cook the whole mixture for about 15 minutes.

- Turn off the heat and let it stand for a few minutes before serving.

Potato Cauliflower and Pea Curry

Total Time: 35 Minutes

Ingredients

- 1 tablespoon vegetable oil

- 1 large shallot, diced

- 4 garlic cloves, finely chopped

- 1 tablespoon fresh ginger, finely chopped or grated

- 1 red chilli pepper, finely chopped

- 1 tablespoon garam masala

- ½ teaspoon turmeric

- ½ teaspoon cayenne pepper

- 1 x 400 g (14 oz) can crushed tomatoes

- 200 g (7 oz) frozen or fresh peas

- 1 small cauliflower head, cut into bite-size florets

- 2 large potatoes, peeled and cubed

- 600 ml (2.5 cups) vegetable stock

- 2 tablespoons fresh coriander, finely chopped

Directions

- Heat the olive oil in a large, heavy-bottomed pot. Sauté the shallot for 2-3 minutes over medium heat until slightly softened.

- Add the garlic, ginger and red chilli pepper and continue to cook for another minute until fragrant.

- Stir in the spices and cook for a further minute, stirring occasionally. Next, add the tomatoes, peas, cauliflower, potatoes and vegetable stock to the pot and bring to a boil.

- Lower the heat and simmer for 15-20 minutes until the potatoes are fork tender. Stir in the fresh coriander and season to taste. Serve with your favourite steamed rice or roti.

Lemon Herb Chicken & Rice

Total Time: 30 Minutes

Ingredients

- 4 boneless skinless chicken breasts

- 2 tablespoons butter

- salt and pepper to taste

- 2 teaspoons Italian seasoning

- 1 cup uncooked white rice

- 2 ¼ cups chicken broth

- juice of 1 lemon

- 1 teaspoon Italian seasoning

Directions

- Melt butter over medium heat in a large skillet or pan (one that has a lid). Season chicken with salt and pepper to taste, and Italian seasoning. Brown chicken in the butter for 1-2 minutes on each side. (Chicken shouldn't be cooked through at this point) Transfer chicken to a plate.

- Add rice, chicken broth, lemon juice, and remaining Italian seasoning to the pan (no need to clean it first). Place chicken on top, then cover and simmer over medium-low heat for 20-25 minutes until liquid is dissolved.

- Garnish with fresh parsley or cilantro if desired and lemon wedges for squeezing. Serve immediately

Total Time: 40 Minutes

Ingredients

- 1 lb. green beans trimmed

- 2 medium sized gold potatoes cubed

- 2 tablespoons olive oil

- 1 teaspoon dried basil

- 1 teaspoon dried oregano

- 1/2 teaspoon garlic powder

- 1 tablespoon butter

- Salt and freshly ground black pepper

Directions

- Bring a large pot of water to boil and add beans. Cook until bright green in color and tender crisp; approximately 2-3 minutes. Plunge cooked beans into a bowl of ice water to stop the cooking process. When completely cool, drain the beans in a colander.

- Place cubed potatoes, olive oil, basil, oregano, and garlic powder in a large bowl and stir to coat. Heat skillet over medium-high heat and add potatoes. Cook until starting to brown, stirring occasionally.

- Lower heat to medium-low so as not to over-brown the potatoes before they are tender. Stir occasionally. Cook until golden brown and tender. Add the well-drained green beans and butter. Season with salt and freshly ground black pepper to taste. Cook for an additional 3-5 minutes.

Total Time: 60 Minutes

Ingredients

- 1 pound sweet potatoes, cut into 1 ¼-inch cubes

- ¾ pound carrots, cut into 1 ¼-inch pieces

- ¾ pound parsnips, cut into 1 ¼-inch pieces

- 1 acorn squash, seeded, cut into 1 ¼-inch pieces

- 1 large red onion, peeled, with root end left intact cut into ½-inch wedges

- ¼ cup extra-virgin olive oil

- 3 tablespoons balsamic vinegar

- 2 tablespoons maple syrup

- 1 tablespoon fresh thyme leaves or rosemary

- Salt and pepper

- Nonstick cooking spray

- Carrot Top Cashew Pesto (optional)

Directions

- Preheat oven to 425°F. Spray an extra-large, rimmed baking sheet (20x15), or 2 large ones (18x12), with non-stick cooking spray.

- Place sweet potatoes, carrots, parsnips, acorn squash, and red onion in a large bowl. Add olive oil, vinegar, syrup, and thyme. Season generously with salt and black pepper. Toss to coat.

- Spread vegetables on prepared pan(s) in a single layer. Roast uncovered 40-45 minutes until vegetables are softened and browned, stirring halfway through.

- Can be made 3 hours ahead. Transfer to clean baking sheet and let stand at room temperature. Rewarm at 375°F for 10-15 minutes. Serve with Carrot Top Cashew Pesto as desired.

Creamy zucchini soup

Total Time: 53 Minutes

Ingredients

- 1 tbsp Coles Classic Olive Oil

- 1 onion, coarsely chopped

- 1 garlic clove, crushed

- 4 large zucchini, chopped

- 2 large potatoes, peeled, chopped

- 1L Massel chicken style liquid stock

- 3/4 cup cream

- salt and cracked black pepper

Directions

- Heat 1 tablespoon oil in a large saucepan over medium heat. Add 1 coarsely chopped onion, 1 crushed garlic clove, 4 large chopped zucchini and 2 large peeled, chopped potatoes. Cook for 5 minutes, making sure vegetables don't brown.

- Add 1L chicken stock and 1 cup water. Bring soup to the boil, reduce heat and simmer for 20 minutes or until potatoes are soft. Remove from heat and cool for 5 minutes.

- Blend with a hand-held blender until smooth. Return soup to the heat and add 3/4 cup cream, salt and cracked black pepper. Warm through and serve with bread or corn and chive mini muffins.

Total Time: 60 Minutes

Ingredients

- 2 tbsp avocado oil, or olive oil

- 1 medium onion, diced

- 3 cloves garlic, minced

- 3 tablespoons ginger, minced or finely diced

- 2 pounds carrots, peeled and chopped

- 4 cups vegetable broth

- 1 bay leaf

- 1 teaspoon cinnamon

- 1 teaspoon salt

- Optional toppings: coconut cream, crispy shallots, toasted pine nuts and cilantro

Directions

- Heat the oil over medium-high heat in a large pot. Add the onions and cook for 1 to 2 minutes or until translucent.

- Add the ginger and garlic to the pot and stir for another minute.

- Place the chopped carrots in the pot and stir to combine. Cook for 10 minutes, stirring often.

- Add the broth, bay leaf, cinnamon and salt to the pot. Bring to a boil, then cover and turn the heat to low for a gentle simmer. Cook for 20-30 minutes or until the carrots are soft when pierced with a fork.

- Turn off the heat and remove the bay leaf. Blend the soup with an immersion blender or transfer the soup to a high-powered blender. Blend the soup until it's pureed and smooth.

- Divide each portion of soup into a bowl. If you'd like, swirl one tablespoon of coconut cream on top and garnish with crispy shallots, toasted pine nuts, and cilantro.

Roasted Chicken and Butternut Soup
Total Time: 55 Minutes

Ingredients

- 4 bone-in, skin-on chicken thighs

- 1 medium butternut squash (about 2 ½ pounds), peeled, seeded, and diced medium

- 1 small yellow onion, diced medium

- 2 tablespoons extra-virgin olive oil

- Coarse salt and ground pepper

- 4 cups low-sodium chicken broth or water

- ¼ teaspoon ground cumin

- ¼ teaspoon ground coriander

- 1 to 2 tablespoons fresh lemon juice

- Fresh cilantro (optional)

Directions

- Preheat oven to 425 degrees. In a roasting pan or rimmed baking sheet, toss together chicken, squash, onion, and oil; season with salt and pepper. Arrange in a single layer and roast until squash and chicken are cooked through, about 30 minutes.

- Transfer chicken to a plate and let cool. Transfer squash and onions to a medium pot and add broth, cumin, and coriander. Bring to a simmer over medium-high. With a potato masher or back of a wooden spoon, mash some vegetables until soup is thick and chunky. Discard skin and bones from chicken; cut meat into small pieces and add to soup. Stir in lemon juice; season to taste with salt and pepper. To serve, top with fresh cilantro, if desired.

Total Time: 55 Minutes

Ingredients

- 4 parsnips

- 2 tablespoon olive or rapeseed oil

- 1 onion

- 2 garlic cloves

- 2 teaspoon curry powder mild or medium

- 750 ml vegetable stock

- 50 ml dairy-free cream

Direction

- Preheat the oven to 180°C / 350°F.

- Peel the parsnips and cut into wedges, and place in a roasting tin or baking tray. Peel the onion and slice thickly and add to the tray, then add the garlic cloves - whole and unpeeled. Drizzle over the oil, add the curry powder and season with salt and black pepper, then toss everything together until the vegetables are fully coated with oil.

- Roast for 30 minutes until the parsnips are golden brown and soft. Remove the garlic cloves (keep them for later), and set aside.

- Bring the vegetable stock to the boil in a large saucepan. Tip in the roasted parsnips and onion, then squeeze the soft flesh out of the roasted garlic cloves, add to the pan and discard the skin. Boil for 4-5 minutes, then remove from the heat, stir through the cream then blitz to a very smooth purée with a hand blender or in a blender / food processor. Taste and adjust seasoning as required.

- If you wish to make parsnip crisps for a garnish, simply peel strips off a parsnip with a potato peeler. Heat a little oil in a frying pan and fry the strips gently until they are just turning golden brown. Watch carefully, they can burn in seconds! Sprinkle with salt then remove from the pan and keep on kitchen paper until just before serving so they stay crisp.

- Serve the soup with a drizzle of cream and your parsnip crisps.

CONCLUSION

HEALTH IS WEALTH! STAY SAFE ALWAYS!!!